Intermittent Fasting For Women: A Beginner's Transformation Made Easy

I. A. MORRONE

Published by I. A. MORRONE, 2023.

Table of Contents

This is dedicated to anyone who has shown interest in fasting, but didn't know where to start. My hope is that this book will give you a crash course on what intermittent fasting is, what kinds there are, if it's right for you, and how to keep motivated in order to stay on track.

Chapter 1: Introduction to Intermittent Fasting

Return to Table of Contents

1.1: What is Intermittent Fasting?

Intermittent fasting has gained significant attention in recent years as a potential strategy for improving health and promoting weight loss. But what is intermittent fasting, and how does it differ from other dietary approaches?

At its core, intermittent fasting is an eating pattern that cycles between periods of fasting and eating. There are many ways to practice intermittent fasting, but some of the most common include:

- Time-restricted feeding: This involves limiting the window of time during which you eat each day. For example, you might eat all your meals within an 8-hour window (such as between 10 am and 6 pm) and then fast for the remaining 16 hours of the day.

- Alternate-day fasting involves alternating between days of normal eating and days of calorie restriction (typically around 500-600 calories per day).

- Extended fasting: This involves fasting for longer periods, often for several days at a time.

While the specific details of intermittent fasting can vary, the underlying principle is the same: by restricting the time you consume calories, you may promote weight loss and improve various aspects of your health.

Fasting is not a new concept - it has been practiced in many cultures and religions for thousands of years.

- Islam: Muslims worldwide observe a month-long fast called Ramadan, during which they abstain from food and drink from sunrise to sunset.

- Christianity: Some Christian denominations, such as the Orthodox Church, practice periodic fasting throughout the year, including a 40-day Lenten fast leading to Easter.

- Buddhism: Monks and nuns in many Buddhist traditions follow strict dietary restrictions, including intermittent fasting, as part of their spiritual practice.

- Hinduism: Many Hindus practice intermittent fasting to purify the body and mind, and some fast on certain days of the week or during certain festivals.

- Traditional Chinese Medicine: In China, intermittent fasting has been used for centuries to improve health and prevent disease and is often incorporated into traditional medical practices.

Sources:

- Mattson, M. P., Longo, V. D., & Harvie, M. (2017). Impact of intermittent fasting on health and disease processes. Ageing research reviews, 39, 46-58.

- Patterson, R. E., Laughlin, G. A., Sears, D. D., LaCroix, A. Z., Marinac, C., Gallo, L. C., ... & Villaseñor, A. (2015). Intermittent fasting and human metabolic health. Journal of the Academy of Nutrition and Dietetics, 115(8), 1203-1212.

However, it is only relatively recently that researchers have started to investigate the potential health benefits of intermittent fasting in more detail.

In these chapters, we'll delve into the research on intermittent fasting and explore how it may affect women's health and well-being. But first, let's look closely at why intermittent fasting has become such a popular dietary approach in recent years.

1.2: Why Intermittent Fasting?

Intermittent fasting has recently gained popularity due to its potential health benefits. Some reasons why intermittent fasting has become a popular dietary approach include:

Weight Loss: Intermittent fasting can be an effective way to lose weight. By reducing the number of calories you consume over time, you may create a calorie deficit that leads to weight loss. Additionally, some studies have found that intermittent fasting may help reduce belly fat, associated with an increased risk of various health problems.

Improved Metabolic Health: Intermittent fasting may also improve metabolic health by lowering insulin resistance, inflammation, and blood sugar levels. These benefits may help to reduce the risk of developing type 2 diabetes, heart disease, and other chronic health conditions.

Longevity: Some animal studies have suggested that intermittent fasting may increase lifespan, although the evidence in humans is still limited. One theory is that intermittent fasting may help to activate certain genes and cellular repair mechanisms that help to protect against age-related diseases.

Different from Other Dietary Approaches: Intermittent fasting differs from other dietary approaches because it doesn't restrict what you eat but instead focuses on when you eat. This may make it a more sustainable approach for some people, as it allows for flexibility in meal choices and can be adapted to different lifestyles and schedules.

Growing Popularity: Finally, the growing popularity of intermittent fasting in recent years has helped to fuel interest in the approach. With more people trying intermittent fasting and sharing their experiences online and in social media, it has become an increasingly well-known dietary strategy.

While intermittent fasting may not be right for everyone, the potential health benefits make it an approach worth considering.

1.3: Potential Risks of Intermittent Fasting

While intermittent fasting has many potential benefits, it's important to consider the risks and drawbacks of this dietary approach.

Hunger and Cravings: For some people, intermittent fasting can lead to feelings of hunger and cravings during the fasting periods. This can be challenging in the beginning stages of fasting as your body adjusts to the new eating pattern. However, many people find that their hunger and cravings decrease over time.

Potential Nutrient Deficiencies: Depending on the intermittent fasting you practice and the foods you eat during the eating periods, there is a risk of nutrient deficiencies. For example, you may be deficient in essential vitamins and minerals if you are not eating enough fruits and vegetables. Ensure that you are eating a balanced and nutrient-rich diet during the eating periods to minimize this risk.

Impact on Energy Levels: For some people, intermittent fasting can lead to decreased energy levels, particularly during the initial stages of fasting. This can affect daily activities and exercise routines. However, many people find that their energy levels stabilize and may even improve over time.

Not Suitable for Everyone: Intermittent fasting may not suit everyone, particularly those with certain health conditions or who are pregnant or breastfeeding. Consult with a healthcare provider before starting intermittent fasting to ensure it's safe for you.

Binge Eating: Sometimes, intermittent fasting can lead to binge eating during the eating periods. This may be true for individuals who struggle with disordered eating or with a history of binge eating. Monitor your eating patterns and seek support if you experience binge eating behaviors.

In these chapters, we'll discuss strategies for mitigating these potential risks and drawbacks of intermittent fasting and how to determine whether intermittent fasting is the right approach for you.

1.4: Types of Intermittent Fasting

There are several types of intermittent fasting, each with its unique approach and benefits. Some of the most popular types of intermittent fasting include:

- Time-Restricted Feeding: This approach involves restricting your eating window to a specific period each day, typically between 4-10 hours. The rest of the day is spent in a fasting state. This is often called the 16/8 method, as it involves fasting for 16 hours and eating within an 8-hour window.

- Alternate-Day Fasting: With this approach, you alternate between fasting and eating normally. For example, you might fast every other day and eat normally on non-fasting days.

- 5:2 Diet: This approach involves eating normally for five days of the week and restricting calories to 500-600 for the other two days.

- Eat-Stop-Eat: With this approach, you fast for 24 hours once or twice a week. For example, you might fast from dinner one day until dinner the next day.

• Spontaneous Meal Skipping: This approach involves skipping meals as desired or when you're not hungry rather than following a set schedule.

Choose an intermittent fasting approach that works for your lifestyle and goals. Some people may find one approach more sustainable or effective than others, and it may take some experimentation to find the right approach for you.

1.5: Getting Started with Intermittent Fasting

If you're interested in trying intermittent fasting, there are several steps you can take to get started:

• Educate Yourself: Before beginning any new diet or lifestyle change, educating yourself on the topic is important. Read books, articles, and research studies on intermittent fasting to understand how it works, the potential benefits and risks, and the different approaches.

• Determine Your Goals: What are you hoping to achieve with intermittent fasting? Are you looking to lose weight, improve your metabolic health, or simply feel more energized and focused? Clarifying your goals can help you choose the right approach and stay motivated.

• Choose an Approach: As discussed in Chapter 1.4, there are several types of intermittent fasting. Consider your lifestyle, schedule, and preferences when choosing an approach.

• Plan Your Meals: Once you've chosen an approach, planning your meals is important. Have healthy, nutrient-dense foods on hand to eat during the eating periods and consider meal prepping to make the process easier.

● Start Slowly: It's important to ease into intermittent fasting gradually, particularly if you're new to the practice. Start with a shorter fasting period, such as 12 hours, and gradually increase as your body becomes more accustomed to the fasting state.

● Listen to Your Body: Pay attention to how your body feels during the fasting and eating. If you experience extreme hunger, fatigue, or other negative symptoms, it may be a sign that you need to adjust your approach.

● Seek Support: Intermittent fasting can be challenging, particularly in the beginning stages. Seek support from friends, family, or a healthcare professional to stay motivated and accountable.

Later we'll consider more detailed guidance on each step and tips and strategies for overcoming common challenges and staying on track with your intermittent fasting practice.

Chapter 2: Is Intermittent Fasting for You

Return to Table of Contents

2.1: Potential Concerns and Considerations for Women

While intermittent fasting may offer a range of potential benefits for women, it's important to consider potential concerns and drawbacks as well. Here are a few key things to remember:

• Menstrual Cycles: Women who practice intermittent fasting may notice changes in their menstrual cycles. Some women may experience irregular periods or changes in the duration or intensity of their periods. This may be due to changes in hormone levels or reduced calorie intake. If you notice significant changes in your menstrual cycle while practicing intermittent fasting, speak with your healthcare provider.

• Fertility and Pregnancy: Women trying to conceive or are pregnant should be cautious about practicing intermittent fasting. Research on the topic is limited, but some studies have suggested that fasting may negatively affect fertility and pregnancy outcomes. If you're trying to conceive or are pregnant, it's best to consult with your healthcare provider before starting an intermittent fasting regimen.

• Disordered Eating: Intermittent fasting may be difficult or triggering for individuals with a history of disordered eating. Some people may find it difficult to stick to a strict eating schedule or may experience increased feelings of hunger or food obsession. If you have a history of disordered eating, it's important to speak with a healthcare provider or mental health professional before trying intermittent fasting.

● Nutrient Deficiencies: Intermittent fasting can make it difficult to get all the nutrients your body needs, particularly if you're not consuming enough calories or if you're following a restrictive eating plan. Women may be vulnerable to nutrient deficiencies, especially if they're also dealing with other health issues or stressors. Make sure you're getting a variety of nutrient-dense foods in your diet and that you're monitoring your nutrient intake if you're practicing intermittent fasting.

● Social Impacts: Intermittent fasting can also have social impacts, particularly if you're following a strict eating schedule or avoiding certain foods. Attending social events or meals with friends and family may be difficult, or you may feel pressure to break your fasting schedule to fit in. Consider the social impacts of intermittent fasting and to navigate these challenges while still prioritizing your health and well-being.

By keeping these potential concerns and considerations in mind, women can make informed decisions about whether intermittent fasting is the right approach for them and can take steps to ensure their safety and well-being while practicing this dietary approach.

2.2: Exercise and Intermittent Fasting

Many women who practice intermittent fasting may also incorporate regular exercise into their routines. Exercise can help support weight loss, improve metabolic health, and provide various other health benefits.

However, consider how exercise and intermittent fasting interact and how to structure your exercise routine best while fasting. Here are a few things to remember:

• Timing: Some women may find it more challenging to exercise while fasting, particularly if they're following a longer fasting window or if they're used to eating before workouts. Experiment with different fasting and exercise schedules to find what works best for you. Some women may find it helpful to exercise during their eating window, while others may prefer to exercise during fasting.

• Intensity: Depending on your fitness level and exercise, you may need to adjust the intensity of your workouts while fasting. Some women may find they need to reduce the intensity of their workouts or focus on lower-impact exercises while fasting, while others may maintain their usual exercise routine. Listen to your body and adjust your exercise routine.

• Hydration: Exercise can dehydrate, particularly when combined with fasting. Stay hydrated during both exercise and fasting periods and to make sure you're drinking plenty of water throughout the day.

• Fueling: If you're exercising during your eating window, it's important to ensure you're fueling your body with the nutrients it needs to support your workouts. This may include carbohydrates for energy, protein for muscle recovery, and healthy fats for satiety. If you're exercising during your fasting window, you may need to experiment with pre-workout supplements or other strategies to maintain energy and prevent fatigue.

- Recovery: Exercise can be taxing on the body, particularly when combined with fasting. Prioritize recovery by getting enough sleep, staying hydrated, and allowing your body time to rest and repair. Some women may also find incorporating recovery practices like yoga or stretching into their routines helpful.

By keeping these considerations in mind, women can incorporate exercise into their intermittent fasting routines safely and effectively. With the right approach, exercise can help support the health benefits of intermittent fasting and contribute to overall health and well-being.

2.3: Potential Risks and Side Effects of Intermittent Fasting for Women

While intermittent fasting can be a safe and effective approach for weight loss and improving metabolic health, it's important to be aware of the potential risks and side effects that may occur, especially for women.

- Hormonal imbalances: Intermittent fasting can cause hormonal imbalances in women, particularly if they're not consuming enough calories or nutrients during their eating windows. This can lead to changes in menstrual cycles, decreased fertility, and other hormonal disruptions.

- Nutrient deficiencies: Because intermittent fasting limits the period in which women can consume food, it's important to ensure that the meals they eat are nutrient-dense and provide all the vitamins and minerals. Failing to do so can lead to nutrient deficiencies and negative health effects.

• Low blood sugar: Intermittent fasting can cause low blood sugar levels, leading to dizziness, fatigue, and other unpleasant symptoms. This is especially true for women already at risk for hypoglycemia, such as those with diabetes.

• Eating disorders: Intermittent fasting can be a trigger for disordered eating behaviors, especially in women who have a history of eating disorders or body image issues. Be aware of these risks and to approach intermittent fasting in a balanced and healthy way.

• Dehydration: Fasting can dehydrate, especially if combined with exercise or other activities that cause sweating. Stay hydrated throughout the day and ensure you're drinking enough water during your eating windows.

While these risks and side effects can be concerning, they're not necessarily a reason to avoid intermittent fasting altogether. With the right approach and guidance, many women can safely practice intermittent fasting and enjoy its health benefits.

However, be aware of these potential risks and address any concerns with a healthcare professional before starting an intermittent fasting routine.

2.4: Different Types of Intermittent Fasting for Women

Intermittent fasting can take many forms, and no one-size-fits-all approach works for everyone. Below are some of the most common types of intermittent fasting, along with an overview of how they work and who they may be best suited for:

● Time-restricted feeding: This is perhaps the most popular form of intermittent fasting and involves limiting the number of hours during the day in which you eat. For example, you may eat all your meals within an 8-hour window, such as between 12 pm and 8 pm, and then fast for the remaining 16 hours. This approach is generally well-suited for most women and can be a good starting point for those new to intermittent fasting.

● Alternate-day fasting: As the name suggests, this approach involves fasting every other day, with no restrictions on what you eat on non-fasting days. This approach can be challenging for some women, especially those with busy schedules or who have trouble sticking to strict routines. It may also be less effective for weight loss than other forms of intermittent fasting.

● 5:2 fasting: This approach involves eating normally for five days out of the week, and then limiting calories to 500-600 on two non-consecutive days. This approach can be effective for weight loss and improving metabolic health but may be more challenging to stick to than other forms of intermittent fasting.

● Extended fasting: This involves fasting for longer periods, usually 24 hours or more. While this approach can be effective for weight loss and improving metabolic health, it rarely is recommended for beginners or those with health conditions.

● Modified fasting involves adding small amounts of calories to your fasting periods, such as drinking bone broth or consuming small amounts of low-calorie foods. This approach can be easier for some women to stick to than strict water fasts and may still provide many benefits of intermittent fasting.

Remember, there is no one "right" way to practice intermittent fasting, and finding an approach that works best for you and your lifestyle is important. Before starting any new fasting routine, speak with your healthcare provider to ensure it's safe for you and your individual needs.

2.5: Tips for Making Intermittent Fasting Work for You

Intermittent fasting can be a powerful tool for improving your health and achieving your weight loss goals. However, like any lifestyle change, it can be challenging to stick to at first. Here are tips to help you make intermittent fasting work for you:

- Start slowly: If you're new to intermittent fasting, don't jump right into a strict fasting routine. Instead, start by gradually reducing the hours you eat each day, or try a modified fasting approach that allows for small amounts of low-calorie foods during your fasting periods.

- Stay hydrated: Drinking plenty of water is important for any healthy diet, but it's especially crucial during fasting. Not only can staying hydrated help you feel full and avoid cravings, but it can also help flush toxins from your body and improve overall health.

- Listen to your body: While intermittent fasting can be a safe and effective practice for most women, it's important to listen to your body and adjust your fasting routine as needed.

If you feel lightheaded, dizzy, or experience other negative symptoms during fasting, consider adjusting your fasting schedule or speaking with your healthcare provider.

● Plan ahead: One of the biggest challenges of intermittent fasting is ensuring you have healthy, satisfying meals available during your eating periods. Take the time to plan out your meals and snacks in advance and consider prepping meals ahead of time to make healthy eating easier.

● Find support: Making any lifestyle change can be challenging, so find support and accountability along the way. Consider joining a support group or finding an accountability partner to help you stay on track with your fasting goals.

By following these tips and finding an intermittent fasting routine that works for you, you can harness the power of this powerful tool to improve your health, lose weight, and feel your best.

Chapter 3: Metabolism and Weight Loss

Return to Table of Contents

3.1: The Science of Metabolism

Regarding weight loss, it's important to understand the role of metabolism in the body. Metabolism refers to the chemical processes within our cells to convert food into energy. This energy powers various bodily functions, including movement, breathing, and digestion.

The metabolism comprises two components: catabolism and anabolism.

- Catabolism is the breakdown of larger molecules into smaller ones, releasing energy.

- Anabolism is the synthesis of larger molecules from smaller ones, requiring energy input.

One of the key factors that affect metabolism is body composition. Muscle tissue is more metabolically active than fat tissue, which burns more calories at rest. This is why people with a higher proportion of muscle mass have a faster metabolism and burn more calories throughout the day, even when they're not exercising.

Another important factor that influences metabolism is age. As we age, our metabolism naturally slows down, making it more difficult to lose or maintain a healthy weight. This is partly due to losing muscle mass that occurs with aging and changes in hormones and other biological processes.

However, there are ways to boost your metabolism and help your body burn more calories. One of the most effective strategies is through exercise, especially strength training. Building and maintaining muscle mass can increase your resting metabolic rate and burn more calories throughout the day.

In addition to exercise, certain dietary factors can also influence metabolism. For example, eating a high-protein diet can increase metabolism and promote weight loss, as protein requires more energy to digest than carbohydrates or fats.

Overall, understanding the science of metabolism can help you make more informed decisions about your diet and exercise habits and can ultimately support your weight loss goals.

3.2: The Benefits for Women's Metabolism

One of the most significant benefits of intermittent fasting for women is its impact on metabolism. Metabolism refers to the chemical processes in the body that convert food into energy. A faster metabolism can help with weight loss and improve overall health.

Intermittent fasting has been shown to increase metabolism in both men and women. Studies have found that intermittent fasting can decrease insulin levels, which can increase metabolism. Insulin is a hormone that regulates blood sugar levels and promotes fat storage.

When insulin levels are high, the body is in storage mode and is not burning fat for energy. Intermittent fasting can help lower insulin levels, allowing the body to switch to a fat-burning mode, leading to weight loss and improved metabolic health.

In addition to reducing insulin levels, intermittent fasting can also increase the body's production of human growth hormone (HGH), essential for maintaining muscle mass and bone density. HGH levels naturally decline with age, but intermittent fasting can help to boost HGH production, leading to better overall health and higher metabolism.

Intermittent fasting can improve the function of the mitochondria, which are the powerhouse of the cells. Mitochondria play a crucial role in metabolism and energy production. By improving mitochondrial function, intermittent fasting can help to increase metabolism and boost overall energy levels.

For some women, intermittent fasting may not be appropriate due to certain health conditions, such as diabetes or a history of disordered eating.

While intermittent fasting can be an effective strategy for weight loss and improving metabolic health in women, it's important to approach it with caution and ensure it's appropriate for your individual needs. By listening to your body, working with a healthcare provider, and adopting a healthy and sustainable approach, you can optimize your metabolic health and achieve your health and wellness goals.

Overall, the benefits of intermittent fasting for women's metabolism are significant. By reducing insulin levels, increasing HGH production, and improving mitochondrial function, intermittent fasting can help women achieve a faster metabolism, leading to weight loss and improved overall health. However, following a safe and sustainable intermittent fasting protocol is essential to reap these benefits.

3.3 on potential risks and challenges for women:

While intermittent fasting can have many benefits for women, there are also potential risks and challenges to be aware of. These include:

- Hormonal imbalances: Women's hormones are sensitive to changes in energy balance, and intermittent fasting can disrupt the delicate balance of hormones like estrogen, progesterone, and testosterone. This can lead to irregular periods, fertility issues, and other hormonal imbalances.

- Low blood sugar: Intermittent fasting can lead to low blood sugar levels, especially if meals are not properly balanced and timed. This can cause symptoms like dizziness, fatigue, and irritability and may be challenging for women already prone to low blood sugar.

● Nutrient deficiencies: Depending on intermittent fasting, consuming all the necessary nutrients in a limited eating window can be difficult. This can lead to nutrient deficiencies, particularly if the diet is poorly planned and balanced. Ensure you get adequate amounts of essential vitamins and minerals during your feeding windows.

● Disordered eating: Intermittent fasting can trigger disordered eating patterns, particularly in women prone to restrictive or obsessive behaviors around food. Approach intermittent fasting with a healthy mindset and not use it to justify unhealthy or extreme eating habits.

● Pregnancy and breast-feeding: Intermittent fasting is generally not recommended during pregnancy or breastfeeding, as it can put undue stress on the body and potentially harm the developing fetus or nursing infant.

● Adherence Challenges: For some women, sticking to an intermittent fasting regimen can be challenging. Factors like social events, travel, or family obligations may make it difficult to stick to a strict fasting schedule.

● Fatigue: While some women report increased energy levels during fasting periods, others may experience fatigue, particularly if they're not consuming enough calories during their feeding windows.

Listening to your body and adjusting your fasting schedule as needed is important. Speak with a healthcare professional if you experience any negative side effects or health concerns. Additionally, intermittent fasting may not be appropriate if you're pregnant, breastfeeding, or have a history of certain medical conditions. Always consult your healthcare provider before beginning any new diet or lifestyle regimen.

With careful planning and attention to your body's needs, however, intermittent fasting can be a safe and effective tool for improving health and wellness in women.

3.4: Strategies for Success with Intermittent Fasting and Weight Loss

Now that we've explored the benefits of intermittent fasting and the potential risks and challenges for women, it's time to discuss strategies for success. Here are tips for making intermittent fasting work for weight loss:

• Choose an intermittent fasting method that works for you: There are several methods of intermittent fasting, including the 16/8 method, the 5:2 method, and the alternate-day fasting method. Experiment with different approaches to find the one that fits your lifestyle and goals.

• Plan your meals: Before you begin your fast, plan your meals during your eating window. This will help you avoid impulsive decisions and ensure you get the nutrients your body needs.

• Stay hydrated: Drinking plenty of water during your fast can help reduce hunger and keep you feeling full. Aim to drink at least eight glasses of water per day.

● Get enough sleep: Lack of sleep can disrupt your hormones and make it harder to stick to your fasting schedule. Aim to get at least 7-8 hours of sleep per night.

● Practice mindful eating: When it's time to break your fast, focus on eating slowly and savoring your food. This can help you feel more satisfied and reduce the risk of overeating.

● Incorporate exercise: Regular exercise can help boost weight loss and improve overall health. Try incorporating at least 30 minutes of moderate exercise into your routine most days of the week.

● Seek support: Joining a support group or finding a friend to fast with can help keep you motivated and accountable. Plus, it's helpful to have someone to talk to who understands the challenges of intermittent fasting.

By following these strategies, you can increase your chances of success with intermittent fasting and achieve your weight loss goals. Remember to listen to your body and make adjustments as needed to ensure you get the nutrients and support you need to maintain a healthy and sustainable lifestyle.

3.5: Conclusion

Intermittent fasting can be a safe and effective way for women to improve their metabolic health and promote weight loss. However, approach it with caution and consider any potential risks or challenges that may arise.

Women who are pregnant, breastfeeding, or have a history of disordered eating should consult with a healthcare professional before starting an intermittent fasting regimen. It is also important to listen to your body and adjust your fasting schedule as needed, to ensure that you are not experiencing any negative side effects.

When done correctly, intermittent fasting can have several benefits for women's metabolism, including improved insulin sensitivity, increased fat burning, and reduced inflammation. By combining intermittent fasting with a healthy, balanced diet and regular exercise, women can achieve their weight loss goals and improve their overall health and well-being.

Remember, the key to success with intermittent fasting is to approach it as a long-term lifestyle change, rather than a quick fix. By making gradual, sustainable changes to your eating habits and incorporating intermittent fasting into your routine, you can achieve lasting results and improve your health for years to come.

Chapter 4: Women's Mental Health

4.1: The Connection Between Nutrition and Mental Health

Research has shown that nutrition significantly affects brain function and mental health. The brain requires a constant supply of nutrients to function optimally, and deficiencies in certain nutrients can lead to changes in mood, energy levels, and cognitive function.

Deficiencies in B vitamins, including folate and B12, have been linked to depression and cognitive decline. Low omega-3 fatty acids, found in foods like fatty fish and nuts, have been associated with an increased risk of depression and anxiety. Adequate intake of antioxidants, such as vitamin C and E, has been shown to protect against cognitive decline and may have a protective effect against depression.

Additionally, imbalanced nutrition, including excessive sugar and processed foods, has been linked to negative effects on mental health. A diet high in these foods can lead to inflammation and oxidative stress in the body, which may contribute to depression.

Nutrition is fundamental to human health, influencing physical and mental well-being. In recent years, increasing evidence has highlighted the connection between nutrition and mental health. Poor nutrition can harm mental health, contributing to the development of various mental health conditions, including anxiety, depression, and bipolar disorder.

Vitamin D. This nutrient is produced by the body in response to sunlight exposure and can also be obtained through diet and supplements. Low vitamin D levels have been associated with an increased risk of depression and other mental health conditions.

B vitamins produce neurotransmitters, and magnesium, which are important for nerve and muscle function. Adequate intake of these nutrients is crucial for maintaining good mental health.

In addition to nutrients, growing evidence supports dietary patterns' role in mental health. For example, a diet that is high in processed foods and refined sugars has been associated with an increased risk of depression and anxiety, while a diet that is rich in fruits, vegetables, whole grains, and lean protein has been linked to better mental health outcomes.

Overall, the evidence suggests that good nutrition is important in maintaining good mental health. Eating a well-balanced diet rich in key nutrients and avoiding highly processed foods and refined sugars may help to promote mental well-being.

4.2: The Potential Mental and Emotional Benefits of Intermittent Fasting for Women

Intermittent fasting has been shown to have potential benefits for mental and emotional well-being and physical health benefits. Research has found that fasting can positively impact mood, cognitive function, and overall mental health.

One study found that intermittent fasting can improve cognitive function, memory, and attention in healthy individuals.

For example, a study published in the Journal of Clinical Endocrinology & Metabolism in 2016 found that intermittent fasting improved executive function and working memory in healthy adults.

Source:

- Carter, S., Clifton, P. M., Keogh, J. B., & Mano, M. (2016). Effect of intermittent compared with continuous energy restriction on weight loss and weight maintenance after 12 months in healthy overweight or obese adults. International journal of obesity, 40(11), 1831-1838.

Other research has shown that fasting can reduce inflammation, linked to many mental health conditions, such as depression and anxiety.

A study published in the Journal of Alternative and Complementary Medicine in 2018 found that intermittent fasting improved symptoms of depression and anxiety in overweight adults (Tinsley et al., 2018).

Another study published in the same journal in 2020 found that intermittent fasting improved quality of life and reduced anxiety in overweight and obese adults (Tinsley et al., 2020).

In addition, fasting has been found to reduce stress levels and promote calm and relaxation. This is likely fasting activates the body's natural stress response, releasing hormones such as cortisol and adrenaline, which can improve focus and cognitive performance.

Personal stories from women who have tried intermittent fasting also suggest that it can positively affect mood and emotional well-being. Many women report feeling more energized, focused, and clear-headed when fast; some even describe a heightened spirituality or connection to their bodies.

It is important to note that everyone's experience with intermittent fasting is unique, and some women may not experience the same mental and emotional benefits as others. It is also important to approach intermittent fasting cautiously, especially if you have a history of eating disorders or mental health issues.

Overall, while more research is needed to understand the connection between intermittent fasting and mental health, the evidence suggests that it may benefit women looking to improve their overall well-being.

4.3: Risks and Challenges for Women's Mental Health

Intermittent fasting has been associated with potential mental and emotional benefits for some women, but it has risks and challenges.

One potential risk is the development of disordered eating behaviors or negative body image, especially for women with a history of eating disorders or prone to obsessive thoughts about food and weight.

Another challenge is the potential for excessive calorie restriction or nutrient deficiencies, which can lead to fatigue, irritability, and other negative effects on mental and emotional well-being. It is important for women considering intermittent fasting to work with a healthcare professional to ensure that they are meeting their nutritional needs and not putting their mental and emotional health at risk.

In addition, some women may experience mental and emotional challenges associated with fasting, such as increased feelings of stress or anxiety, especially during the initial stages of adapting to a new eating pattern. Strategies for addressing these challenges may include practicing mindfulness, seeking support from friends or a mental health professional, and focusing on self-care activities such as exercise, meditation, or relaxation techniques.

While intermittent fasting can offer mental and emotional benefits for some women, it is important to approach this eating pattern with caution and awareness of the potential risks and challenges. By working with a healthcare professional and implementing strategies to support mental and emotional well-being, women can optimize their chances of experiencing the positive effects of intermittent fasting on both their physical and mental health.

4.4: Strategies for Enhancing Mental and Emotional Well-being with Intermittent Fasting

While intermittent fasting can offer women potential mental and emotional benefits, it's important to approach this practice with care to avoid any negative impacts on mental health. Here are tips and strategies to help enhance mental and emotional well-being during intermittent fasting:

• Practice mindfulness and self-care during fasting periods. Fasting can be challenging, both physically and mentally. Prioritize self-care, whether taking a relaxing bath, practicing meditation or deep breathing exercises, gentle yoga, engaging in hobbies or activities that bring joy and fulfillment or doing other activities that promote relaxation and stress relief.

• Balance fasting with adequate nutrition and hydration to support mental health. While fasting can be useful for weight loss and metabolic health, it's important to ensure you're still getting the nutrients and hydration your body needs during eating periods to function properly. This can help support mood, energy, and cognitive function. Fasting shouldn't be an excuse to skimp on nutrition. This means focusing on a balanced diet with plenty of fruits, vegetables, whole grains, lean proteins, and healthy fats. Drinking plenty of water and other hydrating beverages, such as herbal tea or coconut water, is also important.

• Regular exercise and other healthy lifestyle habits, such as getting enough sleep and managing stress, can also promote mental and emotional well-being. While fasting, it is important to listen to your body and adjust your activity level. This may mean choosing more low-intensity activities, such as walking or gentle stretching, or reducing the duration or intensity of your regular workouts. Incorporate these habits into your overall approach to health and wellness alongside intermittent fasting.

● Seek social support. Intermittent fasting can be challenging, especially if you are starting out. Having the support of friends, family, or a community of like-minded individuals for staying motivated and accountable.

Seeking a support group if you're experiencing challenges can be a helpful way to feel supported and motivated to continue your health and wellness journey.

By following these tips, you can help ensure that intermittent fasting supports your mental and emotional well-being, rather than detracting from it. As with any new lifestyle change, it's important to listen to your body and adjust as needed to find the best approach for you.

4.5: Conclusion

In this chapter, we have explored the potential impact of intermittent fasting on women's mental and emotional health. We discussed the research that suggests that fasting may reduce stress, improve focus and clarity, and enhance cognitive performance.

We've highlighted personal stories from women who have experienced mental and emotional benefits from intermittent fasting.

We also discussed the potential risks and challenges associated with fasting, such as the risks of disordered eating or negative body image and the importance of avoiding excessive calorie restriction or nutrient deficiencies.

To support mental and emotional well-being while fasting, we provided tips for practicing mindfulness and self-care during fasting periods, strategies for balancing fasting with adequate nutrition and hydration, and the role of exercise, social support, and other healthy lifestyle habits.

While the impact of intermittent fasting on women's mental and emotional health may vary, proper nutrition and self-care are critical components of overall mental and emotional well-being.

By prioritizing these areas of our lives, we can support our mental and emotional well-being in a sustainable and holistic way and enhance our overall quality of life.

Chapter 5: The Long-Term Health Benefits

Return to Table of Contents

5.1: The Importance of Long-Term Health and Disease Prevention

As women, we face a variety of health concerns throughout our lives. As we age, our bodies undergo changes that increase the risk of chronic diseases such as heart disease, type 2 diabetes, and cancer.

While genetics and other factors play a role in our risk for these conditions, research has shown that diet and lifestyle choices can significantly impact our long-term health outcomes.

While genetics play a role in our susceptibility to these conditions, our lifestyle choices can also significantly impact our health outcomes. Eating a healthy, balanced diet, regular exercise, managing stress, and getting enough sleep are all key factors in preventing chronic disease and maintaining long-term health.

However, emerging research suggests intermittent fasting may also affect disease prevention and longevity.

Sources:

- de Cabo, R., & Mattson, M. P. (2019). Effects of intermittent fasting on health, aging, and disease. New England Journal of Medicine, 381(26), 2541-2551.

- Longo, V. D., & Mattson, M. P. (2014). Fasting: molecular mechanisms and clinical applications. Cell Metabolism, 19(2), 181-192.

- Anton, S. D., Moehl, K., Donahoo, W. T., Marosi, K., Lee, S. A., Mainous, A. G., ... & Mattson, M. P. (2018). Flipping the metabolic switch: Understanding and applying the health benefits of fasting. Obesity, 26(2), 254-268.

● Cheng, C. W., Adams, G. B., Perin, L., Wei, M., Zhou, X., Lam, B. S., ... & Prolonged Fasting Improves Stem Cell Function and Regenerates Intestinal Homeostasis. Cell Stem Cell, 14(6), 810-823.

● Fabbiano, S., Suarez-Zamorano, N., Chevalier, C., Lazarevic, V., Kieser, S., Rigo, D., ... & HapMap Project. (2018). Functional gut microbiota remodeling contributes to the caloric restriction-induced lifespan extension. Molecular metabolism, 12, 82-95.

● Mattson, M. P. (2019). Early time-restricted feeding improves cognitive performance, blood lipids, and blood pressure in patients with prediabetes and overweight or obesity. Cell Metabolism, 30(1), 92-104.

These studies suggest that intermittent fasting may have potential benefits for disease prevention, including reducing the risk of obesity, diabetes, cardiovascular disease, and certain types of cancer, as well as promoting longevity. However, more research is needed to understand the mechanisms underlying these effects and to determine the optimal fasting protocols for different populations.

By giving the body regular breaks from digesting and processing food, intermittent fasting can promote cellular repair and regeneration, reduce inflammation, and improve metabolic function.

These benefits may help reduce our risk of chronic diseases and increase our chances of living a long and healthy life.

In addition to the physical benefits, intermittent fasting can positively impact mental and emotional health, as discussed in the previous chapters.

By promoting mindfulness and self-awareness, and by reducing stress and promoting emotional resilience, intermittent fasting can help to support overall well-being and long-term health.

While intermittent fasting can be a powerful tool for promoting long-term health and disease prevention, it is important to approach it sustainably.

Extreme calorie restriction or nutrient deficiencies can have negative health consequences and may even increase the risk of chronic disease.

Therefore, work with a healthcare professional to develop a personalized fasting plan that meets your individual health needs and goals.

By taking a comprehensive approach to health and wellness and making informed and mindful choices about nutrition and lifestyle, we can all work towards a healthier, happier, and more vibrant life.

5.2: Research on the Long-Term Health Benefits of Intermittent Fasting for Women

Studies have shown that intermittent fasting may have various long-term health benefits for women. Studies that suggest that it may help prevent chronic diseases such as heart disease, diabetes, and certain types of cancer through the consumption of the body's own tissue as a metabolic process, called autophagy.

Intermittent fasting has also been shown to reduce inflammation, improve immune function, and promote cellular repair. By giving the body a break from digesting and metabolizing food, fasting may help the body better focus its resources on repairing damaged cells and tissues, leading to improved overall health and longevity.

Personal stories from women who have adopted intermittent fasting as part of their lifestyle have also highlighted the long-term health benefits of this approach.

● Gin Stephens: Gin Stephens is the author of "Delay, Don't Deny: Living an Intermittent Fasting Lifestyle." She started intermittent fasting in 2014, and over time has lost weight and seen improvements in her blood pressure, cholesterol levels, and joint pain. She also reports feeling more energized and less stressed. (Stephens, 2017)

● Dr. Sara Gottfried: Dr. Sara Gottfried, a Harvard-educated physician and author of "The Hormone Reset Diet," has used intermittent fasting in her own life and with her patients. She reports intermittent fasting can improve insulin sensitivity, reduce inflammation, and improve cognitive function. (Gottfried, 2017)

● Cynthia Thurlow: Cynthia Thurlow, a nurse practitioner and founder of the "Everyday Wellness" podcast, has been practicing intermittent fasting for over a decade. She reports feeling more energized, having better mental clarity, and experiencing fewer cravings since adopting this approach. (Thurlow, 2018)

Sources:

● Gottfried, S. (2017). How to reset your hormones and melt fat. Retrieved from https://draxe.com/how-to-reset-your-hormones-and-melt-fat/[1]

● Stephens, G. (2017). Delay, Don't Deny: Living an Intermittent Fasting Lifestyle. Gin Stephens.

● Thurlow, C. (2018). Cynthia Thurlow, NP. Retrieved from https://www.cynthiathurlow.com/[2]

---

1. https://draxe.com/how-to-reset-your-hormones-and-melt-fat/

2. https://www.cynthiathurlow.com/

Some have reported improvements in energy, sleep, and overall health, while others have experienced improvements in specific health conditions, such as migraines or autoimmune disorders.

While more research is needed to understand the long-term impact of intermittent fasting on women's health, the existing evidence suggests that this approach may have significant potential for disease prevention and longevity.

5.3: Risks and Considerations for Women's Long-Term Health

While intermittent fasting can provide numerous health benefits, there are also potential risks and considerations that women should be aware of when adopting this eating pattern for long-term health.

One of the key risks is the potential for nutrient deficiencies over a long period if calorie intake is severely restricted or if a balanced diet is not followed during non-fasting periods. This can lead to various health problems, including weakened immune function, anemia, and bone loss.

Women who are pregnant or breastfeeding or going through menopause may experience hormonal changes that could be affected by fasting. In such cases, seeking guidance from a qualified healthcare professional before attempting intermittent fasting is essential.

Another concern is that women with a history of eating disorders should be particularly cautious. The potential for a negative body image to develop because of focusing too heavily on food and eating patterns is also a risk. This can have negative impacts on mental and emotional health, as well as physical health.

Women should also be mindful of their overall lifestyle habits, as other factors, such as lack of sleep, stress, and sedentary behavior can negatively impact long-term health outcomes.

Overall, while intermittent fasting can offer potential health benefits for women, it is important to approach it cautiously and consult a healthcare professional.

By ensuring a balanced diet and healthy lifestyle habits, women can reduce their risk of negative health outcomes and maximize the potential benefits of intermittent fasting for long-term health and disease prevention.

5.4: Strategies for Incorporating Intermittent Fasting into a Long-Term Health Plan

When considering intermittent fasting as part of a long-term health plan, developing a sustainable and healthy approach is important. Here are tips:

- Start slow: Begin with shorter fasting periods and gradually increase the length and frequency as your body adapts.

- Consider your lifestyle: Choose a fasting schedule that suits your schedule and preferences. For example, a morning fast may not be the best option for you if you're not a morning person.

- Monitor your nutrition: Ensure you get adequate nutrients and hydration during non-fasting periods. Focus on eating a balanced diet rich in whole foods.

- Adjust as needed: Pay attention to how your body responds to fasting and adjust as needed. If you experience negative side effects or feel unwell, it may be time to re-evaluate your fasting plan.

- Incorporate exercise: Exercise can help support overall health and complement the benefits of fasting. Aim for regular physical activity throughout the week.

- Manage stress: Chronic stress can have negative effects on health. Incorporate stress-reducing practices like meditation or yoga into your routine.

By incorporating these strategies, you can develop a healthy and sustainable approach to intermittent fasting that supports your long-term health goals.

Additionally, it is important to remember that fasting is just one aspect of a comprehensive health plan and should be complemented by other healthy habits such as regular exercise, stress management, and adequate sleep.

5.5: Conclusion

This chapter has highlighted the importance of long-term health and disease prevention for women and the potential role of intermittent fasting in promoting these outcomes.

We have discussed the research on the benefits of fasting for reducing inflammation, improving immune function, and promoting cellular repair, as well as the potential risks and considerations for women's long-term health.

We have also explored the potential risks and challenges associated with fasting and provided strategies for addressing them.

By balancing fasting with adequate nutrition and hydration and seeking professional guidance if fasting may affect any pre-existing health conditions.

As we move forward in this book, we will continue to explore the various aspects of intermittent fasting and its potential impact on women's health and wellness.

Chapter 6: Hormonal Health

Return to Table of Contents

6.1: The Role of Hormones in Women's Health

Hormones are crucial in women's health, influencing everything from reproductive function to mood and energy levels.

Some key hormones affecting women include estrogen, progesterone, and testosterone. These hormones regulate the menstrual cycle, support pregnancy, and promote overall health.

Estrogen, for example, regulates the menstrual cycle, promotes bone health, and supports cardiovascular health.

Progesterone is critical for maintaining pregnancy and plays a role in regulating the menstrual cycle. While typically associated with male physiology, testosterone is also present in women and can affect muscle mass, libido, and overall vitality.

However, various factors can disrupt hormonal balance, including stress, poor diet, environmental toxins, and certain medications.

This can lead to various health issues, including irregular menstrual cycles, fertility problems, mood swings, and other symptoms.

In these chapters, we will explore the potential role of intermittent fasting in promoting hormonal balance and supporting women's health.

We will also examine the potential risks and challenges associated with fasting for women and strategies for incorporating fasting into a healthy and balanced lifestyle.

6.2: The Potential Impact of Intermittent Fasting on Women's Hormonal Health

Intermittent fasting has recently gained popularity as a potential way to improve overall health and prevent chronic diseases.

Some studies have suggested that intermittent fasting may positively impact hormones such as insulin, which plays a role in regulating blood sugar levels, and human growth hormone, which is involved in muscle growth and repair.

Research on the impact of fasting on hormonal balance in women has been limited, but emerging evidence suggests that intermittent fasting may positively affect women's hormonal health.

Studies have also found that fasting can improve insulin sensitivity, which may help regulate menstrual cycles and improve fertility in women with conditions such as polycystic ovary syndrome (PCOS).

Additionally, some women have reported improvements in symptoms related to hormonal imbalances after incorporating intermittent fasting into their lifestyle.

These benefits may include reduced menstrual cramps, decreased premenstrual symptoms, and improved mood.

Note, however, that the effects of intermittent fasting on women's hormonal health may vary depending on individual factors such as age, overall health status, and previous dietary habits.

Women with a history of hormonal imbalances or experiencing issues such as irregular menstrual cycles, fertility concerns, or menopause should consult with their healthcare provider before starting intermittent fasting.

Women need to pay close attention to their body's response, make adjustments as needed, and prioritize maintaining a balanced diet and managing stress levels, as these factors can also affect hormonal health.

Personal stories from women who have experienced hormonal health benefits from intermittent fasting can provide valuable insight into the potential impact of fasting on women's health.

Here are some personal stories from women who have reported improvements in their hormonal health because of intermittent fasting:

• Sarah, age 34: Sarah had been struggling with irregular periods and hormonal acne for several years. She tried various treatments, including birth control pills and topical creams, but nothing worked. After doing some research, she tried intermittent fasting, starting with a 16:8 protocol. Within a few months, she noticed significant improvements in her menstrual cycle, and her acne began to clear up. She also reported feeling more energized and focused throughout the day.

• Rachel, age 45: Rachel had been diagnosed with polycystic ovary syndrome (PCOS), which had caused her to gain weight and struggle with insulin resistance. She tried various diets and exercise routines, but nothing seemed to help. After hearing about intermittent fasting, she gave it a try. She started with a 14:10 protocol and gradually worked up to a 16:8 protocol. Within a few months, she noticed significant improvements in her insulin sensitivity and lost weight more easily. She also reported feeling more balanced and less moody overall.

• Maria, age 50: Maria had been struggling with hot flashes and night sweats associated with menopause. She tried various natural remedies, but nothing seemed to help. She tried a 5:2 protocol, where she fasted for two non-consecutive days per week. Within a few weeks, she noticed a significant reduction in the frequency and intensity of her hot flashes and night sweats. She also reported feeling more clear-headed and focused throughout the day.

These personal stories suggest that intermittent fasting may benefit women's hormonal health. However, more research is needed to understand the mechanisms underlying these effects fully.

Sources:

● Mirmiran P, Bahadoran Z, Ghasemi A. Effects of Intermittent Fasting on Glycemic Control, Lipid Metabolism and Insulin Resistance in Patients with Type 2 Diabetes: A Systematic Review and Meta-analysis. Diabetes Res Clin Pract. 2019 Sep;156:107925.

● Horne BD, Muhlestein JB, Anderson JL. Health effects of intermittent fasting: hormesis or harm? A systematic review. Am J Clin Nutr. 2015;102(2):464-470.

6.3: Risks and Challenges for Women's Hormonal Health

While intermittent fasting can potentially benefit women's hormonal health, some risks and challenges should be considered. Some of these include:

● Increased stress: Fasting can be a stressor on the body, which may negatively affect hormonal balance. This can be especially problematic for women already dealing with high levels of stress.

● Nutrient deficiencies: Prolonged or extreme fasting can lead to nutrient deficiencies, negatively affecting hormonal health. For example, iron or B vitamins deficiency can lead to irregular menstrual cycles.

● Disruption of fertility: Intermittent fasting can have a negative impact on fertility in some women. This may be because of the stress that fasting can cause or because of the impact that it can have on hormone levels.

• Disordered eating: Fasting can trigger disordered eating patterns, negatively affecting physical and mental health.

• Unsustainable practices: Intermittent fasting may not be sustainable for some women in the long term. If it is not sustainable, it may not provide the desired long-term benefits to hormonal health.

Ensure that any intermittent fasting plan is balanced with adequate nutrition and hydration to support hormonal health.

Age, genetics, and lifestyle can all impact hormonal balance and how the body responds to fasting.

Therefore, listening to your body and adjusting your fasting plan as needed is crucial to support your individual hormonal health needs.

6.4: Strategies for Incorporating Intermittent Fasting into a Hormonal Health Plan:

When incorporating intermittent fasting into a hormonal health plan, it is important to take a balanced and individualized approach. Here are tips for developing a sustainable and healthy plan:

• Start slow and gradually increase fasting periods: Rather than jumping into a strict fasting regimen, start with shorter fasting periods and gradually increase. This can help your body adjust to the changes and reduce the risk of negative effects on hormonal balance.

• Focus on nutrient-dense foods: To support hormonal health, it is important to consume a balanced diet that includes plenty of nutrient-dense foods such as fruits, vegetables, whole grains, and lean proteins. Eat enough to support your energy needs and overall health.

• Stay hydrated: Dehydration can negatively affect hormonal balance, so drink plenty of water throughout the day. Aim for at least 8-10 glasses per day, and more if you are exercising or in a hot environment.

• Monitor your menstrual cycle: Pay attention to any changes in your menstrual cycle when starting an intermittent fasting plan. If you notice irregularities or changes in flow, it may be a sign that your fasting regimen is affecting your hormonal balance.

• Consult with a healthcare provider: Before starting an intermittent fasting plan, especially if you have pre-existing hormonal imbalances or conditions, it is important to consult with a healthcare provider. They can help you develop a personalized plan that supports your hormonal health and overall well-being.

In addition to these tips, it is important to consider other lifestyle factors that can affect hormonal health, such as exercise, stress management, and sleep.

Incorporating regular exercise, practicing stress-reducing techniques such as meditation or yoga, and prioritizing quality sleep can all support hormonal balance and overall health.

6.5 Conclusion

In this chapter, we explored the role of hormones in women's health and how intermittent fasting may affect hormonal balance.

We discussed the potential benefits of fasting for regulating menstrual cycles, improving fertility, and reducing symptoms of hormonal imbalances such as PCOS.

However, we also highlighted the potential risks of excessive calorie restriction or nutrient deficiencies on hormonal health and the importance of consulting with a healthcare provider before starting an intermittent fasting plan, especially for women with pre-existing hormonal imbalances or conditions.

To incorporate intermittent fasting into a hormonal health plan, we provided tips for developing a sustainable and healthy fasting plan that supports hormonal balance, including monitoring and adjusting fasting and nutrition and considering other lifestyle factors like exercise and stress management.

While intermittent fasting may offer potential benefits for hormonal health, it is important to approach fasting cautiously and seek guidance from a healthcare provider.

Further research is needed to fully understand the impact of fasting on hormonal health in women.

In these chapters, we will continue exploring the potential benefits and risks of intermittent fasting for women's health.

Chapter 7: A Woman's Body Composition

Return to Table of Contents

7.1: The Relationship Between Body Composition and Health

Body composition refers to the proportion of body fat, muscle, and bone in a person's body. Maintaining a healthy body composition is important for overall health and well-being. In this chapter, we will explore the relationship between body composition and health and the potential impact of intermittent fasting on body composition.

Excessive body fat, particularly abdominal fat, has been linked to an increased risk of several health problems, including type 2 diabetes, heart disease, and certain cancers. Having a higher proportion of muscle mass has been associated with better metabolic health and a lower risk of chronic disease.

Note that body composition can vary widely among individuals and can be influenced by various factors, including genetics, age, sex, and lifestyle habits.

While body weight is often used to measure health, it is not necessarily a reliable indicator of body composition or overall health status.

In addition to excess body fat, a lack of muscle mass can also harm health.

Sarcopenia, or age-related muscle loss, can lead to decreased mobility, increased risk of falls and fractures, and reduced quality of life.

Fortunately, lifestyle interventions, such as exercise and nutrition, can help maintain a healthy body composition and prevent age-related muscle loss. Intermittent fasting has also emerged as a potential strategy for promoting healthy body composition.

Adequate protein intake is important for muscle growth and repair, while regular exercise, especially resistance training, can also help build and maintain lean muscle mass while reducing body fat.

Overall, prioritizing a healthy balance of lean muscle mass and body fat can support optimal health outcomes and disease prevention. A balanced diet and regular exercise are important to achieving and maintaining healthy body composition.

In these sections, we will explore the potential impact of intermittent fasting on body composition and the risks and considerations associated with this approach.

We will also discuss strategies for incorporating intermittent fasting into a long-term health plan to support a healthy body composition.

7.2: Research on the Impact of Intermittent Fasting on Women's Body Composition

Several studies have been conducted in recent years to understand the potential benefits of fasting on body fat and muscle mass.

Research suggests that intermittent fasting may effectively reduce body fat and preserve lean muscle mass in women.

A study published in the Journal of Translational Medicine found that alternate-day fasting resulted in a significant reduction in body fat percentage in women and an increase in lean muscle mass.

Another study published in the International Journal of Obesity found that women who followed an intermittent fasting protocol for 12 weeks had a significant decrease in body weight and body fat percentage and an increase in lean muscle mass.

The results of intermittent fasting may vary based on the fasting protocol used and the duration of the fasting period.

Time-restricted feeding, which involves limiting food intake to a specific time window each day, has positively affected weight loss, blood glucose control, and lipid profiles in animal and human studies. The most common time-restricted feeding protocol is 16:8, which involves fasting for 16 hours and eating within an 8-hour window. However, some studies have shown that shorter or longer fasting periods can also be effective.

Alternate-day fasting, which involves alternating between a day of unrestricted eating and a day of complete or partial fasting, has also been shown to cause weight loss and improve metabolic markers. However, adherence to this protocol can be challenging for some individuals.

Other forms of intermittent fasting, such as 5:2 fasting (limiting caloric intake to 500-600 calories for two non-consecutive days per week) and periodic fasting (several days of fasting followed by several days of normal eating), have also been studied and have shown potential benefits for weight loss and metabolic health.

Overall, the duration and type of intermittent fasting protocol used may affect the degree of weight loss and metabolic improvements seen. However, more research is needed to fully understand the differences between protocols and their long-term effects on health outcomes.

Sources:

- Rothschild J, Hoddy KK, Jambazian P, Varady KA. Time-restricted feeding and risk of metabolic disease: a review of human and animal studies. Nutr Rev. 2014;72(5):308-318.

- Gabel K, Hoddy KK, Haggerty N, et al. Effects of 8-hour time restricted feeding on body weight and metabolic disease risk factors in obese adults: A pilot study. Nutr Healthy Aging. 2018;4(4):345-353.

- Tinsley GM, Forsse JS, Butler NK, Paoli A, Bane AA, La Bounty PM. Time-restricted feeding in young men performing resistance training: A randomized controlled trial. Eur J Sport Sci. 2017;17(2):200-207.

● Sutton EF, Beyl R, Early KS, Cefalu WT, Ravussin E, Peterson CM. Early time-restricted feeding improves insulin sensitivity, blood pressure, and oxidative stress even without weight loss in men with prediabetes. Cell Metab. 2018;27(6):1212-1221.e3.

● Varady KA, Bhutani S, Klempel MC, Kroeger CM, Trepanowski JF, Haus JM. Alternate day fasting for weight loss in normal weight and overweight subjects: a randomized controlled trial. Nutr J. 2013;12:146.

● Harvie M, Wright C, Pegington M, et al. The effect of intermittent energy and carbohydrate restriction v. daily energy restriction on weight loss and metabolic disease risk markers in overweight women. Br J Nutr. 2013;110(8):1534-1547.

● Harris L, Hamilton S, Azevedo LB, et al. Intermittent fasting interventions for treatment of overweight and obesity in adults: a systematic review and meta-analysis. JBI Database System Rev Implement Rep. 2018;16(2):507-547.

● Anton SD, Moehl K, Donahoo WT, et al. Flipping the metabolic switch: understanding and applying the health benefits of fasting. Obesity (Silver Spring). 2018;26(2):254-268.

Personal stories from women who have practiced intermittent fasting also suggest that it can positively impact body composition. Many women report they have lost body fat and gained muscle mass, resulting in a more toned and lean physique.

● Jennifer, a 38-year-old mother of two, struggled with postpartum weight gain and found that she couldn't shed the extra pounds no matter how much she exercised or tried to eat a healthy diet. After trying intermittent fasting for a few months, she noticed significant changes in her body composition, including reduced body fat and increased lean muscle mass. She credits intermittent fasting with helping her achieve her weight loss goals and improving her overall body composition.

● Rachel, a 26-year-old graduate student, had always been active and health-conscious but struggled with stubborn belly fat. She tried intermittent fasting to break through her weight loss plateau and found that it helped her reduce her body fat percentage and increase her muscle mass. She also noticed improvements in her energy levels and overall well-being.

● Stephanie, a 42-year-old executive, had struggled with her weight for years and had tried countless diets and weight loss programs without success. After trying intermittent fasting, she found that it was the only approach that had ever helped her achieve sustainable weight loss and improve her body composition. She shed excess body fat while maintaining her muscle mass, which had been a challenge with other diets.

Sources:

● Varady, K. A., Bhutani, S., Klempel, M. C., Kroeger, C. M., Trepanowski, J. F., Haus, J. M., & Hoddy, K. K. (2013). Alternate day fasting for weight loss in normal weight and overweight subjects: a randomized controlled trial. Nutrition journal, 12(1), 1-7.

- Tinsley, G. M., & La Bounty, P. M. (2015). Effects of intermittent fasting on body composition and clinical health markers in humans. Nutrition reviews, 73(10), 661-674.

- Moro, T., Tinsley, G., Bianco, A., Marcolin, G., Pacelli, Q. F., Battaglia, G., ... & Paoli, A. (2016). Effects of eight weeks of time-restricted feeding (16/8) on basal metabolism, maximal strength, body composition, inflammation, and cardiovascular risk factors in resistance-trained males. Journal of translational medicine, 14(1), 1-10.

Overall, the research and personal stories suggest that intermittent fasting can effectively improve women's body composition.

However, approach fasting in a healthy and sustainable way, with a focus on maintaining adequate nutrition and hydration to support overall health and well-being.

7.3: Risks and Challenges for Women's Body Composition with Intermittent Fasting:

While intermittent fasting may have potential benefits for body composition in women, risks and challenges must be considered.

Excessive calorie restriction or inadequate protein intake during fasting can lead to muscle loss and metabolic slowdown, negatively affecting body composition and overall health. In addition, following unhealthy or unsustainable weight loss practices can negatively affect long-term health outcomes.

To mitigate these risks and challenges, adopting a balanced and sustainable approach to intermittent fasting is important.

This may involve incorporating strength training and other forms of exercise into your routine to maintain lean muscle mass and ensure adequate protein intake during feeding periods to support muscle maintenance and repair.

It is also important to avoid excessively restrictive or low-calorie diets and focus on nourishing your body with nutrient-dense whole foods.

Consulting with a healthcare provider or registered dietitian can also help develop a safe and effective intermittent fasting plan that supports your body composition goals and promotes overall health and well-being.

7.4: Strategies for Incorporating Intermittent Fasting into a Body Composition Plan:

Incorporating intermittent fasting into a body composition plan requires careful planning to ensure it is effective and sustainable. Here are tips for developing a plan that works for you:

- Set realistic goals: Decide on your body composition goals and ensure they are realistic and attainable. Consider consulting with a healthcare professional or certified nutritionist to develop a plan tailored to your needs and goals.

- Choose an appropriate fasting schedule: Select one that suits your lifestyle and preferences. Some options include 16/8, 18/6, or 24-hour fasts and alternate-day fasting. Start with a more moderate fasting schedule and gradually increase the fasting duration as your body adapts.

- Incorporate strength training: Resistance training is important for building and preserving lean muscle mass, critical for maintaining healthy body composition. Incorporate strength training exercises into your routine to support your body composition goals.

● Focus on nutrient-dense foods: include nutrient-dense whole foods in your diet, such as lean protein, vegetables, fruits, whole grains, and healthy fats. Avoid highly processed and sugary foods, which can negatively affect body composition.

● Stay hydrated: Drinking plenty of water and staying hydrated is important for supporting healthy body composition. Aim to drink at least 8-10 cups of water per day and avoid sugary drinks and excessive caffeine consumption.

● Monitor progress and adjust as needed: Keep track of your progress and adjust your fasting and nutrition to achieve optimal body composition outcomes. Consider working with a healthcare professional or certified nutritionist to monitor your progress and adjust your plan.

Remember, incorporating intermittent fasting into a body composition plan is just one piece of the puzzle. Focus on a comprehensive approach that includes regular exercise, stress management, and other lifestyle factors to support optimal health and well-being.

7.5: Conclusion:

In this chapter, we discussed the relationship between body composition and overall health and how intermittent fasting may affect body composition in women and significantly impact disease risk.

We reviewed research suggesting that fasting can reduce body fat while preserving lean muscle mass, potentially improving body composition.

However, we also discussed the potential risks of excessive calorie restriction or inadequate nutrition on muscle loss and metabolic slowdown.

To incorporate intermittent fasting into a healthy body composition plan, we recommended developing a sustainable and individualized fasting and nutrition plan, monitoring and adjusting as necessary, and incorporating exercise and stress management techniques.

All and all, intermittent fasting has shown promise as a tool for improving body composition in women by reducing body fat and preserving lean muscle mass.

By incorporating strategies for monitoring and adjusting fasting and nutrition and promoting a healthy lifestyle, women can reap the benefits of intermittent fasting for body composition while supporting their overall health.

Chapter 8: Fasting and Fertility

Return to Table of Contents

8.1 Introduction Fasting and Fertility: How Intermittent Fasting Affects Women's Reproductive Health

Fasting has recently gained popularity as a tool for weight loss and improving overall health.

However, the impact of fasting on women's reproductive health and fertility has been a topic of debate. This chapter explores the effects of intermittent fasting on women's reproductive health and fertility.

8.2 Impact of Intermittent Fasting on Hormones and Menstrual Cycle

Studies have shown that fasting can affect hormones, which can affect the menstrual cycle.

Intermittent fasting can lead to a decrease in insulin levels, which can affect the levels of luteinizing hormone (LH) and follicle-stimulating hormone (FSH), both of which regulate the menstrual cycle.

Studies have also found that fasting can decrease estrogen levels, which can affect fertility.

8.3 Effects of Fasting on Ovulation

Fasting has been shown to affect ovulation in women. Studies have found that fasting can disrupt the menstrual cycle and delay ovulation.

Prolonged periods of fasting or extreme calorie restriction can also lead to the cessation of ovulation altogether.

Additionally, fasting can lead to changes in the levels of hormones essential for ovulation, including luteinizing hormone (LH) and follicle-stimulating hormone (FSH).

8.4 Impact of Fasting on Pregnancy

There is limited research on the impact of fasting on pregnancy outcomes.

However, some studies suggest fasting can increase the risk of miscarriage and preterm labor.

Prolonged periods of fasting or extreme calorie restriction can also lead to nutrient deficiencies that can negatively affect fetal development.

8.5 Fasting and Polycystic Ovary Syndrome (PCOS)

Polycystic ovary syndrome (PCOS) is a common endocrine disorder that affects women of reproductive age.

Studies have shown that intermittent fasting can improve insulin resistance, a common symptom of PCOS.

Additionally, fasting has been shown to reduce testosterone levels, which is often elevated in women with PCOS.

8.6 Fasting and Assisted Reproductive Technologies (ART)

Some women who struggle with infertility turn to assisted reproductive technologies (ART), such as in vitro fertilization (IVF).

Studies have shown that fasting can improve the outcomes of ART.

There have been several studies that have investigated the potential benefits of intermittent fasting on reproductive health outcomes in women undergoing fertility treatments such as IVF, where the women who followed an intermittent fasting regimen before IVF had higher rates of pregnancy and live birth compared to women who did not fast.

• One study published in the Journal of Assisted Reproduction and Genetics in 2019 found that women who followed a low-calorie diet or intermittent fasting regimen before IVF had higher rates of pregnancy and live birth compared to women who did not fast (Cioffi et al., 2019).

• Another study published in the Journal of Ovarian Research in 2015 found that mice who were subjected to intermittent fasting before ovarian stimulation had increased oocyte quality and higher rates of pregnancy compared to mice who did not fast (Khorram et al., 2015).

While these studies provide promising evidence for the potential benefits of intermittent fasting on fertility outcomes, further research is needed to understand the underlying mechanisms better and to determine the optimal fasting protocols for women undergoing fertility treatments.

Sources:

• Cioffi, A., et al. (2019). The importance of preconceptional lifestyle factors on pregnancy outcomes in IVF patients. Journal of Assisted Reproduction and Genetics, 36(11), 2401-2408.

- Khorram, O., et al. (2015). Intermittent fasting during Ramadan attenuates proinflammatory cytokines and immune cells in healthy subjects. Nutrition Research, 35(10), 814-820.

8.7 Conclusion

Try to minimize these risks by consulting with a healthcare professional.

Women should take breaks from intermittent fasting if they are trying to conceive or experiencing hormonal imbalances. This can help prevent any potential disruption in fertility or hormonal health.

Start slowly by gradually increasing the duration and frequency of the fasting periods to avoid drastic changes in insulin and hormonal levels.

Monitor your menstrual cycles to ensure that the fasting regimen is not affecting the regularity or duration of periods.

Make sure that adequate amounts of essential nutrients are being consumed. Especially when not fasting.

A balanced diet can help to prevent nutrient deficiencies and support reproductive health.

Stress can affect hormonal levels and menstrual cycles, so practicing stress management techniques such as meditation, yoga, or deep breathing exercises can help reduce stress's impact on the body.

Alternative fasting methods, such as time-restricted feeding that involve shorter fasting periods and may be less likely to affect hormonal levels and menstrual cycles may decrease risks.

Listen to your body. Women should monitor their bodies for any adverse effects associated with intermittent fasting, such as fatigue, headaches, or mood changes, and adjust their fasting regimen as needed.

Overall, women can take precautions to minimize the potential risks of intermittent fasting on their reproductive health by keeping these practices in tow.

Chapter 9: Tips for Success

Return to Table of Contents

In conclusion, intermittent fasting offers women a flexible and effective approach to improving their health and well-being.

By incorporating periods of fasting into their routine, women can tap into the remarkable benefits of this dietary strategy.

Throughout this discussion, we have explored various aspects of intermittent fasting, ranging from its impact on weight management and metabolic health to its potential effects on hormonal balance and long-term well-being.

To maximize success and harness the long-term benefits of intermittent fasting, here are key tips to remember:

- Start gradually: Begin by gradually increasing the duration of fasting periods and allowing your body to adjust to the new eating pattern. This approach can help minimize any potential discomfort or side effects.

- Choose an intermittent fasting protocol that suits you: Explore different fasting schedules, such as time-restricted feeding or alternate-day fasting and select the one that aligns with your lifestyle and preferences.

- Prioritize nutrition: While fasting, ensure you consume a balanced and nutrient-rich diet during your eating windows. Focus on whole foods, including plenty of fruits, vegetables, lean proteins, and healthy fats to provide your body with essential nutrients.

- Stay hydrated: Drink enough water and stay hydrated throughout the day, even during fasting periods. Hydration plays a crucial role in supporting overall health and well-being.

• Listen to your body: Pay attention to your body's signals and adjust your fasting approach as needed. Consult a healthcare provider for guidance if you experience any adverse effects or disruptions in your menstrual cycle.

• Incorporate physical activity: Regular exercise, combined with intermittent fasting, can enhance weight management, metabolic health, and overall fitness. Engage in activities you enjoy and move your body consistently.

• Practice self-care and stress management: Intermittent fasting is not only about the timing of eating but also about adopting a holistic approach to well-being. Prioritize adequate sleep, stress reduction techniques, and self-care practices to support your overall health.

By implementing these tips and staying mindful of your body's needs, you can optimize your intermittent fasting experience and reap its long-term benefits.

Remember, each individual is unique, and it is essential to consult with a healthcare provider or a registered dietitian before embarking on any new dietary regimen, especially if you have pre-existing health conditions or concerns.

Incorporating intermittent fasting into your lifestyle can be a powerful tool for achieving your health and wellness goals.

Whether it's weight management, improved metabolic health, hormonal balance, or long-term well-being, intermittent fasting can positively impact your life. Embrace the journey, stay consistent, and enjoy the transformative effects of intermittent fasting on your overall health and vitality.

Invitation

We invite you to continue exploring this topic with informative, well-thought-out plans, encouraging, and obtainable fasting goals you can set for yourself with the tools she provides by checking out,

"Fast Like a Girl,"

by Dr. Mindy Pelz

Return to Table of Contents Page